Liebestraum

Stephen Evans

For Daisy

Book Layout ©2017: BookDesignTemplates.com

Liebestraum /Stephen Evans – 1st Edition

ISBN: 978-1-7345135-7-8

Prologue

Liebestraum Number 3 by Franz Liszt was one of the first songs I learned to play on the piano. *Liebestraum* in German means a dream of love. Liszt was inspired by a poem by Ferdinand Freiligrath, which begins O lieb, so lang du lieben kannst (Love as long as you can).

The piece was also my grandmother Daisy's favorite, though the version I learned was a simplified one for beginning students. Daisy was a wonderful piano player, far better than I, though she played entirely by ear. I can imagine the concerts they had before my grandfather died, she on the piano and he on the violin.

Daisy (Nana to me) lived with my family for the last few years of her life. When I would play *Liebestraum*, she would come and sit on the piano bench next to me and listen. When she died, she left her piano to me, a gift I will always treasure.

She didn't need to close her eyes as she listened; she was nearly blind at the time. She endured blindness with the fortitude that characterized her life. It was only after she died that I learned some of the story of her life and the hardships she endured during the Depression and after, and came to admire her so.

Daisy loved as long as she could. This book is dedicated to her, and the family she gave us.

Harpman

On November 1, 2005, my brother Michael died. He was a six-foot-six Brad Pitt lookalike, smart, wickedly funny, played the blues harmonica, and was more wholly himself than anyone I have ever met. I can't remember him ever being sick until the cancer took him.

At his wake, I read this:

> *I have been thinking a lot recently about time. How fifty years seems like a long time. But fifty years with my brother seems like a moment.*

> *And now we have time. And he has no time.*

> *It took me a while to realize what that means. He is beyond time. Where he is, there is only always.*

> *So it's not that we will be together again, some day. We are together now. As we have always been together. As we will always be together.*

And where he is, it's always a good time.

When I got home, I began to put the finishing touches on my novel *The Marriage of True Minds*. And I wanted something of him to be in the book. So I turned the reading into a story called *The Island of Always*.

It's my favorite part of the book.

My Dream in Chicago

(This is the dream I had after Mike's funeral, my last night in Chicago.)

I was in an office, after hours. It was an open space, one large room with square pillars and lots of empty desks that had been cleared off. I was looking out two large windows in the front of the office on either side of the door. In the distance, there were very tall buildings but I didn't recognize the skyline.

Lots of people were standing around talking. I didn't recognize anyone else except one guy scowling in the corner for some reason (I used to work with him - hadn't thought of him for years- don't know why he was there). We were all waiting. It was a birthday party. I knew that.

After a few seconds, Mike walked in through the front door. He was completely healthy, beyond healthy. His weight was back, and his strength, and his hair. And there was a brightness coming from him. He was himself again.

He was dressed up, but in a way I hadn't seen for years, a camel hair jacket and sweater vest - something he might have worn in high school. Perfect fit -- very sharp - very cool.

After only a few seconds, he said: "I have to go." We weren't surprised. It seemed natural that he had to leave.

Then he said: "I'll see you soon."

Then he went out the door. I lost sight of him. The party went on. We were glad he was able to stop by.

Bowie Court

The tall oak by the swing set

in the corner of the yard,

by the chain link fence that marked

the beginning of beyond,

is there still.

STEPHEN EVANS

Pets

I've never had a pet. I have written books centered around animals and animal rescue, so that it may seem odd. But not owning a pet doesn't mean I haven't known any.

I did have a few tropical fish I had when I was about ten; they didn't seem to enjoy being petted. I tried to build a terrarium in our backyard a few years later, a home for the abundant neighborhood snakes and turtles. Unfortunately it leaked and had to be abandoned, much to the distress of my mother who now had a cement-lined dead leaf collector behind her house.

All my life I have had allergies, which exacerbate my asthma. When I was young, the asthma was serious, keeping me out of school for long periods. I am still very allergic to cats and horses, and mildly allergic to dogs. I like animals, including horses (though I don't know any), cats, and dogs.

My Dad loved dogs. All of them. Any breed. Any age. Anywhere. If you crossed his path with a dog, you had to stop and let him pet your pet. It was not optional.

It seems odd that I don't know if he had a dog when he was young, but I assume he must have. He was born in Callender, Iowa, in the early 1920s and grew up in nearby Fort Dodge. My grandfather had different jobs during those times, but his brothers ran the family farm. I have a picture of it over my desk: white farmhouse and nearby garage flanked by a brick red barn and other structures.

He worked on the farm as a boy and cared for the animals there. But I can't remember him mentioning a dog. I might have learned on his last visit to Iowa; we planned to go and visit the farm. But he had a minor stroke and ended up in the hospital overnight, so we never did get to go.

I suspect his relationship with animals was different back then. His nickname was Trapper, because he was, actually running a trapline for extra money. In Depression-era Iowa, everyone chipped in to get by.

When I was two, we moved from an apartment in Bethesda, Maryland, to a house on Bowie Court in Rockville. The house had a pretty large backyard with a chain-link fence. And back behind that, when we moved anyway though not now, was the Woods. We called it the Woods, because it was as close to forest as we had seen.

Almost as soon as we moved there, we got our first dog, Lucky.

Lucky, who, it turns out, wasn't so much, was a hound of some sort, with a light colored short-haired coat with dark beige patches. Or maybe I just remember that from the old black and white films. Lucky either bit someone or got distemper and was sent to the farm – at least that's what they told the five-year-old me.

Somewhere in that time, we got our one and only cat, Midnight, also the only female other than my mother who ever shared our home (there was Dad, Mom, and, shortly after we moved, four boys). She was a large cat, shiny black with a startling white patch on her throat. She was with us for a few years, and then disappeared, of her own volition I think, possibly uncomfortable with the gender imbalance. I suspect this period was when we learned about my cat allergy.

A few years later there was Pal. If Lucky's tenure was short, Pal's was long – seventeen years – 1964– to 1971. Pal was a beagle and came to us as a Christmas present through my uncle Jim. He was only a few months old, and tiny, not much bigger than my hand (my hand now, not then).

Pal was another hound, true-blooded, and loved to run. He would take any opportunity to get outside. He could easily jump the fence in the back yard if we let him go. Once in a while Dad would take him up in the woods behind our house and just let him go. We would hear him baying far in the distance, throaty and full and pure, one of the purest sounds I have ever heard.

Pal was clever and devious in making his escapes. When my grandmother Daisy came to live with us, she became his primary target. Pal would hide behind the couch in the family room. When she opened the door, he would dart out before she (or likely anyone) could move. Out and away. No one could catch him then. "Oh that devil," she would say.

But he always came home to us. In fact, he became famous for it. In 1967, we moved from one side of Rockville to the other. And when Pal escaped over there, we would call our neighbors at Bowie Court to be on the lookout. Sure enough an hour or two later he would come trotting up the hill to our old house. Though one time he got away and was not so lucky. He must have been hit and dragged by a car, and barely made it home. He took months to recover, but finally was running like before.

Pal was a family present, but he was Dad's dog. For years, after we moved to our new house, Pal would go into the living room around 6:25 and stand looking out the front window, waiting for my father to come home from work at 6:30.

My brother Michael had two dogs: Rufus, a sheepdog lab mix, and Grendel, a german shepherd. They were both wonderful but with completely different personalities. Rufus was an eighty-pound bouncing ball. and Grendel was calm and the sweetest dog I ever knew. Both ended up with in my father's care.

Rufus came to stay with my Dad when Michael went wandering, his version of walkabout. For much of the time I was growing up, Michael was – somewhere, was all we knew. We would hear from him – sometimes he stayed in one place for a while. But finally he would move on.

After several years, Rufus became ill. My older brother DuWayne took him to the vet, who said the pain was severe and advised euthanasia. My brave brother stood by and held Rufus till the end.

Michael finally returned and settled on a boat in Annapolis, which maybe gave him the feeling that he could leave anytime he wanted to, which at that point was enough for him. He found Grendel abandoned in a storm and took her home. She was named after the character in the John Updike book, the monster who wasn't.

Both Rufus and Grendel, large dogs, were terrified of storms. Rufus would try to burrow behind something, usually tipping it over in the process. And Grendel would get as close as possible to my Dad and shiver during the entire storm.

Grendel like many large dogs had dysplasia, and eventually couldn't get on and off the boat without pain and difficulty. So she too came to live with Dad and a deep friendship formed. My father all his life was an early riser, and each morning he would take Grendel out to the golf course for a walk. Grendel would lie patiently outside the clubhouse, greeting the golfers walking to the first tee, as Dad played cards inside. Then they would travel home again.

During Grendel's tenure, I got married, moved away, got divorced, moved home. After the divorce, I stayed for a while with my parents. By that time Grendel's dysplasia had worsened. Her bed had been in my parent's bedroom for years, but now she could no longer handle the stairs.

I was sleeping in the rec room in the basement. So at night I would walk Grendel outside around the back of the house to the basement door. Eventually even that was too much for her; her legs would go out on the slippery back slope. So I would pick her up and carry her down the stairs. She was a big dog, but somehow we managed and when I deposited her in her bed, she seemed content.

Finally her legs gave out all together and she could not stand, could not go on her walks with Dad. She stopped eating and was in constant pain, and though her gentle expression gave little sign, I imagined her psychic pain was deeper.

Or maybe I didn't imagine it. Maybe I knew somehow. If you have a personality, you are a person. Doesn't that seem right? Grendel, and Rufus, and Pal and Midnight and even poor Lucky all had personalities. They were persons to us. And family members.

This time Michael was the brave brother called in to stop the suffering. My father never got over the loss. He told me after that he would never have another dog. And he never did, though he did not lose any opportunity to appropriate anyone else's.

I was thinking today how the loss of a 'pet' may be deeper in some ways than other losses, because it is less complicated. A marriage or most any human relationship is so complicated that the loss is complicated too. But the relationship with a pet is so much simpler, and the loss so intense.

And yet maybe easier to heal for that same reason. The love is pure, the loss pure, but the memories are pure as well. For Dad, the loss never disappeared. It's just the love and the memories overwhelmed it.

I don't know for sure.

I've never had a pet.

Gene

My father, 87 and victim of a debilitating stroke and dementia, still finds joy in life, in a good meal, a good movie (anything with John Wayne), Burger King, any passing dog, but most in his wife of 63 years whose name he cannot remember. In his sons he finds comfort and aid and laughter.

His eyes still shine with the familiar humor, though often only he understands the joke. His courage inspires me every day, and I am more proud than I can say to be his son.

Eulogy

"There are these two golfers. They're on the tee getting ready to hit when one of them spots a funeral procession going by. So he takes off his hat and holds it over his heart. And the other golfers says "you know, that was really nice –- that was really thoughtful". The first golfer puts his hat back on and says "well, she was a good wife for 25 years..."

That was one of Dad's jokes. He was the best storyteller I ever knew, but his signature phrase was "I just tell 'em; I don't explain 'em".

You all probably know that he was an Iowa farm boy who joined the Navy and moved east to marry my mother, that he was a salesman and manager at General Electronics on Wisconsin Avenue, and for many years a member at Redgate golf course in Rockville.

Some things you might not know: His nickname was Trapper, because as a young man he ran a trapline in Iowa. In the Navy during WWII, he served on troop transports in the North Atlantic. He loved to sing, and had a fine tenor voice and wonderful talent for harmony that I didn't inherit. He studied journalism for a bit at George Washington University and was a talented writer, which I hope I did inherit. He could do long long arithmetic calculations in his head, and he made us do them at the dinner table when we were growing up. He was retired for almost as many years as he worked.

And he found so much joy in life. He loved John Wayne movies, Swiss steak, golf –playing and watching, big band music, any dog, keno and scratchoffs, walking, Louis L'Amour, Burger King, Barbra Streisand, lefsa, English history, his friends, his family (immediate and extended), and most of all my mother, his wife of 63 years. When his illness took one joy away, he simply found even more joy in the rest. His courage and grace in these last few years inspired us every day.

We have been imagining the scene in Heaven when he got there: his mother Alma baking pies; his father Ray and my brother Mike discussing the best fishing spots; his buddy Dave dealing the cards; but first to greet him I imagine the dogs, Pal baying in the distance, Rufus with a tennis ball in his mouth, and Grendel curling quietly at his feet.

I'm going to paraphrase Dad a bit here:

> *There are these two golfers in heaven.
> While they are waiting to hit they see this
> guy on the tee with long hair and a beard
> and he swings and hits the ball out of
> sight, a country mile. One golfer says "who
> does he think he is, Jesus Christ?" And the
> other golfer says "He is Jesus Christ, he
> thinks he's Gene Evans".*

Enjoy Heaven, Dad. We'll miss you.

STEPHEN EVANS

Proof

When I walked into the grocery store near my home a few days ago, I had the strongest memory of my father. In the morning, I would drop him at the store and he would walk up and down each aisle to get his daily exercise, then head down to the wine and cheese shop next door to play Keno and buy lottery tickets. Then I'd take him home before heading to work. This was our routine most days for about two years.

Though I have a skeptical inclination, the feeling of him in the store was so strong I wondered if it was a sign. So I walked down to the wine and cheese store myself and bought two lottery tickets, one each for the Megamillion and Powerball prizes. I decided that if I hit both, I would consider that proof of the afterlife.

Well, I did.

Okay, not the jackpots. But I did hit both the Megamillion Gold ball and the Powerball Red ball. The odds of hitting the Gold ball are 1 in

75. The odds of hitting the Red ball are 1 in 62. The odds of hitting both are...well, if I knew enough math to tell you that, I probably wouldn't be playing the lottery. But it's proof enough for me.

So thanks, Dad.

I'll let you know next time I hit Vegas.

At Peter's Gate

"I cannot let you in," he said,
As I half-knew he would.
I could have lived a better life.
In fact, I knew I should.

"No no, not that," he said and smiled,
"Though you are not the first.
You didn't do your best but then,
You didn't do your worst.

"It's just, you've left your soul behind
On earth. So we'll defer.
Just take a seat, we'll chat a while
And wait for her."

Catch and Release

I came to stay with my mother and father because the house where I was living was being painted. I planned to stay for three weeks. I really didn't understand until I was there how much my parents needed care–they seldom asked for help with anything–and had no clue how much they were going to need. But I did have a premonition at the time that I would never leave. So far that has come true.

On occasion, bugs or spiders would get into their home and dealing with them of course was my job. But I wouldn't kill our stray guests. Instead I would try and catch them and relocate them outside.

I had a large plastic cashew jar (empty of course), which I kept ready for the purpose, and I would tear off the back of a magazine to use as the top. I'd cover the visitors with the jar, slide the paper under it, and dash for the door.

Spiders and bugs went out the back door into the tiny garden. If it was summer, I'd drop them on the rose bush or the azalea. If it was winter, I'd place them on the mulch, so they could burrow in against the cold. Mosquitoes went out the front door, hopefully never to bother us again.

I got pretty good at it. Occasionally I lost one on the way and had to perform the feat all over again. Spiders and bugs were pretty easy, though it was delicate work. But grasshoppers were fast and tricky, and the crickets of course would taunt me from their hidden sanctuaries. But I was persistent.

Dad, a former Iowa farm boy whose nickname was Trapper, was continually amused by my no-kill philosophy. But he was also supportive, and we soon formed a catch-and-release partnership.

He delighted in scoping out the carpet in the living room or the hallway and pointing out targets, then watching me stalk them, jar at the ready, and carefully transport them to one venue or another. But as his condition accelerated in the last year of his life, he had trouble distinguishing between a real bug and any dark image on the floor. So he would point out anything he spotted.

"It's just a piece of lint, Dad," I would say more often than not.

Then his eyes would sparkle, and his smile would broaden. And I would smile back. Maybe he knew that it was lint and was joking with me. I was never sure and he couldn't tell me. His language skills had faded. But his humor never did.

A friend has told me that as people near the end of their lives, they begin to separate from this world and participate in the next. I sometimes had the impression that my father had found some deep knowledge that he wished he could share. It may have been a profound awareness of the world to come, or of this world and the life he had lived. Or maybe the knowledge was simply how for the rest of my life a piece of lint on the floor could make me smile.

Sometimes when you catch, you don't release.

Gene Evans World Famous Trapper Sandwich

As they say, when the legend becomes fact, print the legend.

According to Legend, the Trapper Sandwich was designed by my father and perfected by Harry at the snack bar at Red Gate golf course. Wherever we went, Dad would instruct the cooks how to make it, down to the last detail. Though in his opinion no one ever matched Harry's handiwork.

For Dad, the making of a Trapper sandwich was an art in which imperfection was unacceptable. First, you need two egg yolks and one egg white. Mix and fry them in butter. Toast two pieces of good multigrain bread and butter them both. When done, place cheddar cheese on top of the eggs, then fold them over so the cheese is inside the eggs. Place the eggs carefully on the toast, and slice diagonally.

There you have breakfast heaven.

And heaven's breakfast.

Slumgullion

When my father retired from the office, my mother retired from the kitchen. That's how Dad took over the cooking. He was happy to do this, I think, since he liked to cook and my mother (though a wonderful cook) did not.

He preferred simple food: pork chops or mini-hamburgers in our antique electric frying pan, or chili in the oven, or home fries, or great northern (not Navy) bean soup with ham cooked in a huge dented steel pot, enough to feed several families. But his favorite meal was Slumgullion.

Slumgullion was Dad's word for his most eclectic concoctions. The recipe for Slumgullion was ever-changing, but it started with whatever was left over in the refrigerator. He might take some fried rice, a baked chicken breast, green peas, and gravy of some sort, then stir and heat together with unguessable spices. Maybe it sounds awful, but he enjoyed it, and I have to say so did most who tried it.

He was always happy cooking. He loved being active, having something to do or some place to go. But I think it was the creative aspect of Slumgullion that pleased him so, the ability to take what you are given and make something unique and wonderful out of it.

Eventually, a stroke took away most of his cherished activities, including making Slumgullion. We did what we could, my brothers and I, but still his life narrowed to a small area and limited opportunities. Yet to his last day, he had an astonishing capacity to find joy in almost anything: taking a ride to the golf course or grocery store, watching an old TV show, even our attempts at recreating his Slumgullion recipes.

I always thought my father made up the word Slumgullion. But a friend recently informed me that it is a real word, one that Edward Abbey used in the title of a book. In Slumgullion Stew, Abbey defines the word this way:

Slumgullion stew is the name of a dish popular among hoboes and other knights of the open road. Into a big pot over an open fire each man throws whatever he has to contribute-a stolen chicken, a hambone, a can of beans, a jar of salsa, an old shoe-anything edible.

That sounds like something my Dad would enjoy. But in his last years at least, Slumgullion was not just a dish, but a way of life. He found his joy wherever he could, and shared it with everyone he could. He was after all his own greatest creation.

My Father the Writer

When I moved to Minneapolis, my father drove up with me. I spent three enthralled days on the road listening to him tell wonderful tales of growing up in Iowa: how he got his nickname (Trapper); every job he ever held; how he met my mother; his time in the Navy during WWII. And how he wanted to be a writer.

After the war, he enrolled at George Washington University to study journalism, though he had to drop out eventually to support his young family. Somewhere packed away, I have the draft of a novel he started. I don't know if there is a genetic component to writing, but his style reminds me a little of mine - quirky, fast, funny. But I could never match his storytelling bravado in person.

For most of his life, he was a constant and intrepid reader of anything from English history to Louis L'Amour to Jean Auel's Earth's Children series (he would have been delighted to know that the last book in the series was coming out). We shared a special passion for adventure stories from the Forties by authors like Frank Yerby and Edison Marshall, Rafeal Sabatini and Harold Lamb. I would comb used bookstores and bring them to him like the lost treasures out of the tales themselves.

He began the long slow descent into that terrible disease dementia some years before my first novel *The Marriage of True Minds* was published in 2008. He was not able to read it, though he seemed so proud when I showed him the published volume. Reading was a great loss to him I know. It had been so much of his life in his long retirement: golf, cards, reading, and my mother—not in that order.

Dad went into the hospital for the last time the day after Thanksgiving in 2009. By that time he had lost all his words. One moment when we were alone together in the hospital, I showed him a page in a book I was writing called *A Transcendental Journey*. The dedication was to him. He made no sound, but his eyes went wide and I truly felt he understood. It was such a small gesture for all he had given me, but I'm glad I was able to do it.

From time to time over his last few years, we talked about writing a book together, about his boyhood days in Iowa. He even started making notes. As I look at them now, the handwriting reflects the slow decline in his condition. I can't make out the last few words. The letters are too shaky.

I would have enjoyed writing that book. And I would have enjoyed reading it. He infused every tale with humor and joy in the telling. I imagine he could have been quite a writer. Instead he gave me the chance to be one.

I guess that's what being a father is all about.

You can read the story he wrote in my book *The Mind of a Writer and Other Fables.* I hope to finish his story someday, before I finish.

Eternity in a Grain of Sand

Both my mother and father suffered from dementia for some years at the end of their lives. It was very hard to watch, to see the confusion and fear it generated. But I found that to the end they could both experience joy, though in different ways.

It seemed so limited to me, the life they had, but those small joys were everything to them. A glass of ginger ale, a cookie, a song, became life changing, because past and future were gone and all their life was now. And if now was joyful, then all was joyful. That was how it seemed to me. A little bit of eternity in a moment of time.

My Father the Singer

The song 'Shenandoah" was just playing on TV, and it reminded me of Dad. It was a favorite of his, and one he used to sing often. It was one of the few he would sing in a baritone range; Dad had a natural light second tenor voice, with the same wide vibrato that I have.

When he was young, he told me he and his brothers used to sing together, Wally playing the piano and singing with Dad, Clint, and Jim. With a little luck they might have ended up like another Iowa quartet, the Williams brothers, who were out and about at the same time. But it was not to be.

The only instrument Dad played was a ukulele that he got for Christmas one year. He was pretty good at it, playing over and over the same ten tunes in the little red chord book that came with it, and singing along with his fluid cheery voice.

Dad loved music, and growing up I would often find him sitting alone in the living room (where no one else was allowed— not even the dog) and listening the Barbra or Judy or Lanie. He would pump his fist slowly to the beat of the smooth ballads he loved. And flouting the rule, I would go sit with him and listen. It was my first musical education.

During the last year of his life, Dad would go through periods of agitation called sundowning. On these difficult days, when I came home from work, I would put on some piano music, pull the wheelchair up next to him, take his hand, and sing. And while I sang, I would pump his hand up and down the way he used to.

After a while he would usually start to sing with me. He didn't know the lyrics (and often I didn't either). But his tone and pitch were as pure as ever. Sometimes he would switch over and harmonize with me, which always astonished me. I could never do that. I have sung a few duets in my time. But none I remember with more fondness and gratitude than those.

All the four boys are gone now. I hope they have picked up where they left off those years ago in Iowa. If so, heaven is surely the sweeter for it.

The Three Pillars of Care

I have been caring for my parents for some years now (my father passed a couple of years ago, so now it is only my mother). I have come to think in terms of the Three Pillars of Care. (Maybe there are seven pillars, as there are for Wisdom. But I only know three).

1) Safety

2) Health

3) Joy

Of these, for her time and condition of life, I often think the last is the most important. And maybe not just for her.

Term Limits

A man was standing outside the grocery store on Easter Sunday taking signatures for a petition on term limits. To me, term limits are like Voting for Idiots (or is that redundant?).

But I could not stay and talk to him. I was at the store buying an Easter card for my mother, who had been med-evaced to the hospital two days before (she's doing well, thanks). But it made me think about term limits in a whole different way.

At age 85, she flew in a helicopter.

At age 53, I published a novel.

I guess it is never too late.

That's the lesson I'm taking anyway.

It is spring after all.

But what (or which or where or whom) is it never too late for?

STEPHEN EVANS

Strength Enough

I was sitting next to my mother at the nursing home today, holding her hand as she went in and out of sleep, and thinking back to the day almost seven years ago when my brother died. Michael was then about the age I am now, and nearly all of his life, he had been bright and strong and healthy and active. But cancer had so quickly taken all of that away.

I don't know what he knew or felt that day; the morphine left no sure expression on his face, or maybe he had already mostly crossed the divide. But I remember my mother sitting by him on the bed, holding his hand, and comforting him with her calm quiet presence, showing no sign of the desolation I knew was inside her. She was eighty years old at the time, a thousand miles from home, and I remember watching her, wondering at the source of her strength and composure. Was it her religion, her belief in family, or as simple as a mother's love for her son?

She doesn't mention him often now, as her own disease works its ravages on her mind and body. I wish I could reach back in time and borrow some of the strength she showed that day, to give her back some measure of the comfort she surely gave to him. I can't. I don't have the power to reach through time that way. But in remembering, maybe there is strength enough.

Peace Comes Dropping Slow

I was with my mother today and we were quiet together, just listening to piano music. She would turn to me every once in a while and her eyes were so clear and peaceful, and it reminded me of this by Yeats:

And I shall have some peace there,

for peace comes dropping slow,

Dropping from the veils of the morning to where the cricket sings;

There midnight's all a-glimmer,

and noon a purple glow,

And evening full of the linnet's wings.

Where is the Sacred?

My mother asked me this today. She has dementia, and often now can't find the word she wants, so she will substitute one that to her has some relation, either by meaning or sound. Or sometimes I think it may be the right word and I just can't understand the context.

"It's here," I said.

Her 88th Birthday

Today she smiled.

STEPHEN EVANS

Mary Alice Evans
World Famous Potato Salad

Ingredients:

5 pound bag red potatoes

1 medium sized white onion

5 or 6 stalks of celery

4 hard-boiled eggs (and two more hard-boiled eggs)

2 cups Hellman's mayonnaise

Yellow mustard

Half a capful apple cider vinegar

Celery seed

Salt

Pepper

Paprika

Instructions:

Peel and boil the potatoes until tender (test with a fork - not soft).

Drain and cool the potatoes.

While the potatoes are boiling and cooling, cut up celery, eggs, and onion.

Chop celery and onions very fine.

When cool, dice potatoes into cubes (cut in big bowl with a thin knife, half inch cubes, so you can mix well).

Dressing:

Mix the mayo and mustard (not too dark).

Add half a capful apple cider vinegar.

Combine:

Put some dressing on the potatoes and mix well.

Add celery and onions with the rest of the dressing.

Add salt and pepper to taste.

Sprinkle celery seed over top.

Sprinkle paprika on top for decoration.

If it gets dry, add a little milk

(Words to live by).

Just a Day

Today, I spent the day with my mother, was actually able to get her to eat, drove home, stopped at the grocery and picked up a few things, walked out to a spectacular sunset, and thought despite the problems that often consume my thinking how lucky I am to have the life I do.

STEPHEN EVANS

Halo

"Margaret?"

Again a few minutes later: "Margaret?"

She was looking up at the ceiling.

"Do you see Marg?" I asked.

"I heard her," my mother said.

Margaret was her sister, my aunt Marg. Despite the fact that they were outwardly so different and had led such different lives, they had been deeply close.

My mother was eight, Margaret was twelve, when my grandfather died in 1932. They were sent away together to relatives in Baltimore while my grandmother tried to find a way to put the family back together in the heart of the Depression. My mother and my aunt had spoken nearly every day since, until Margaret passed away a decade ago.

My mother doesn't remember now that Marg is gone. When she is distressed she still calls out for her, just as I imagine she did eighty years ago in Baltimore. She wasn't distressed now; she looked peaceful. But she heard something.

I walked out of the nursing home later that night and looked up to see a halo around the moon. It reminded me of another haloed moon, one I had spoken of at Marg's funeral:

Some people are so authentic in our lives that they change us completely just by being who they are. Marg was like that. Many of us probably can't conceive what our life would have been like without her. I certainly can't.

Marg was something different for everyone. She was a funloving friend, a lifelong companion, a devoted aunt and loving sister, a tireless caretaker, and any stray or wild animal's best friend. She loved wacky gifts and wayout gadgets. She could fix your boat, your car, or your watch. She was always what you needed, when you needed it. And she was always herself.

For me, she was a guide. We had many adventures exploring little creeks and inlets up and down the Patuxent in her CrisCraft, or hunting for fossils up at Calvert Cliffs. At night, we would camp out at the Little Beach, light a driftwood fire, and explore the universe, talking for hours about stars and planets and spaceships and alien abductions and anything else we could imagine.

Her endless curiosity ignited mine. When I was seven, she gave me a book on Einstein's Theory of Relativity. Forty years later, that book is one of my most cherished possessions, because it started me on my lifelong adventure of trying to understand everything I could about everything there is. That's how she did it: she changed you by being who she was and sharing herself with you.

When we left the hospital the last night, the moon was full and brilliant as a lighthouse. The clouds were wispy and very high, and there was a crystal halo around the moon. And I thought to myself: there she goes, exploring again, getting ready to guide us on the next adventure.

I stood outside the nursing home and gazed at the hazy moon. "Not yet," I thought.

I didn't hear a response.

Maybe she did.

The Little Beach

There was nothing there but Summer.

STEPHEN EVANS

Melmelmel

Mom: Let's make some words.

Me: I'd love to.

Mom: Melmelmel

Me: Does that mean water flowing over rocks?

(which was on the video we were watching).

She shrugs.

Me: It does now.

STEPHEN EVANS

Peace

I was sitting outside on my porch today reading for a few hours. All during that time birds came visiting. First there was a beautiful jay, stunning blue and quiet for once, nestled into a spot in the sun just a few feet away. Then a robin. Then a few grosbeaks. Some sparrows. Dad's favorite wren who lives in the azalea next door. A woodpecker on the nearby tree. Others I couldn't name. And now there is a doe settled in the shadowed grass about 100 feet away, testing the breeze, with a young buck standing close. Just living. All just living.

Was that so hard, Life?

STEPHEN EVANS

His First Miracle

My mother has been a devout Catholic all her life, not just the going to church kind (which she was) or the making her kids go to Sunday school kind (which she definitely was) but the good works every day visiting the sick and elderly because that is who you are kind.

So when I heard that a new pope was going to be announced I rushed to the nursing home to turn on the TV for her. I did so just before the announcement "habemus papam".

She was highly agitated, not unusual for that time of day, and seemed unable to focus even as the new Pope Francis came out to address the assembled physical and virtual masses. She glanced up as he started speaking then turned away. But after he gave his first blessing, she immediately quieted, and soon fell calmly to sleep.

A miracle? Possibly.

A blessing? Definitely.

STEPHEN EVANS

The Way of Life

Mom and I were watching a DVD today, one of her favorites, a beautiful young woman singing beautiful songs in beautiful settings. Every once in a while Mom would wave to the singer.

I felt a burst of sadness to know her condition had reached a point where she doesn't know the woman on the television isn't real. And yet it gave me joy to see her joy in watching, joy enough to prompt her wave as the beautiful young woman seemed to approach.

This is the way of life, joy and sadness so intertwined we can hardly tell the difference.

Dedication

My novel *The Marriage of True Minds* is dedicated to my aunt Margaret. The dedication reads:

> *Finally, this story would not have been written without the inspiration and encouragement of my aunt Margaret Norris. This book is dedicated to her memory.*

The first sentence was an understatement. Let me explain.

My mother's older sister, Marg had an extraordinary influence on my life. When I was growing up, I spent many summer weeks with her at her place near the Chesapeake in southern Maryland. We shared many things, but mostly a blazing curiosity about pretty much everything. At night, camping on the beach with a driftwood fire, we talked Einstein and aliens, forests and fossils.

Later in life, we didn't spend much time together. I became busy with work, marriage, divorce, life. I would see her on birthdays and holidays. Somehow our connection never waned.

In December 1999, just before Christmas, she went in the hospital. On Christmas Eve, we learned that she had pneumonia. On New Year's Eve, just a few days before her eightieth birthday, we found out that she also had lung cancer. Family members took turns staying with her at her house in southern Maryland and caring for her, two weeks at a time, getting her back and forth to doctors and chemotherapy. I took the first turn.

I was happy to have this time with her. And she was happy I was there. But she was also very worried that I was taking care of her instead of working (something which didn't concern me at all). That she could worry about me given her condition tells you much about her.

So to keep her from worrying, I told her I was writing something. I wasn't really. But I had written a few things before, a play, some stories, so it wasn't *completely* unbelievable. I didn't like to tell her something that wasn't true. But I didn't want her to worry.

On my next turn to care for her, she mentioned again that she was worried about me and work.

So I told her again: I was writing something. I even broke out my laptop once in a while and tried to look busy.

Still she worried. And she was not ever one to let things go. So, I decided that by the next visit I had to have something to show her.

I can never remember her without a dog in her life, even if she had to borrow the neighbor's. And the squirrels and birds of the area worshiped her generosity, I'm sure. She often donated to animal welfare groups. I came across a magazine at her house from an organization named Best Friends, an animal sanctuary in Utah. The magazine had printed a letter from actress Rene Russo documenting the millions of animals each year who are euthanized in animal shelters. I had no idea this horrific situation existed, and couldn't get it out of my mind.

So when my caregiving shift was over and I went home, I began writing a screenplay about a divorced couple, where one of them becomes quixotically dedicated to animal rescue. I wrote the first draft in three weeks.

By my next visit, she was beyond a nephew's care. But I was able to give her a copy of the screenplay. I don't know if she read it (given her condition, I suspect not). But I think she was happy to see it. About a month or so after, she passed away. At the funeral, I began her eulogy with this:

> *Some people are so authentic in our lives that they change us completely just by being who they are. Marg was like that. Many of us probably can't conceive what our life would have been like without her. I certainly can't.*

That screenplay became the basis for *The Marriage of True Minds,* my first novel. I would not have written it without this experience, I believe, and possibly, would not be writing at all without her influence. For a long while, I considered the story her gift to me, the last of so many. But now I think: a gift, yes, a great gift. But not the last.

Great Hearts

My grandmother had a beau.

Beau was Daisy's term, a word from her girlhood. I don't know when she met Gorton, though they both lived in Baltimore in the early 1900s. There is a picture of them standing together on a slim wooden bridge leading over a creek. From their outfits, that period seems right. Daisy, four years older than Gorton, was born on July 7, 1884.

Daisy, my mother's mother, married my grandfather Edgar sometime between 1900 and 1910. Edgar died in 1933. Daisy's father sent her a letter after Edgar's death:

> *Dear Daisy,*
>
> *The news of Edgar's sudden death was a great shock, one that has filled our hearts with deep sorrow and Alice and I extend to you our deepest sympathy...Daisy we fully realize how much you will miss him,*

never have we seen a love for a man greater than yours for Edgar's.

After Edgar died, Daisy went to work at the Hecht Company in downtown Washington DC. She worked there in the Infants department until her retirement, supporting my mother and her other daughter Margaret as they grew (my uncles Jim and Bud were already grown and working).

For many years, Daisy lived with my aunt Marg in their apartment on Wisconsin Avenue in Washington DC. I loved to visit her there. My playground was the National Cathedral across the street. And sometimes we would ride the streetcar across town, for an adventure visiting the Franciscan Monastery and National Shrine, where she usually bought me a medal of one saint or another.

Sometime in the sixties, Daisy and Marg moved to my hometown of Rockville, Maryland, when the building they'd lived in for forty years was sold to developers. My elementary school lay mid-way between their apartment on Talbott Street and our home on Bowie Court. By then Daisy was almost completely blind, as a blood vessel had burst behind her optic nerve some years earlier. I became her seeing-eye kid, guiding her everywhere, including the communion rail at church on Sunday.

Sometimes I would walk to their apartment after school, and 'Nana' and I might stroll down to the nearby shopping center, or even across on Rockville Pike to McDonald's for milkshakes. How a blind woman and an eight-year-old survived that frenzied rush hour traffic is something of a minor miracle.

In the grand expedition of my youth, one afternoon Daisy and I walked the mile and a half from her apartment to my house. Mid-way, across from my school, she sat down on the curb to rest for a bit. But the curb was so low, she couldn't get up. I was taller than she even then, but much lighter. I stood and pulled and she tried and tried but even together we could not get her to her feet. Soon we both started laughing so hard, I had to sit back down again. So we just sat together on the curb, watching the cars pass. Some while later, we finally got control of ourselves, and got her to her feet. Somehow we made it the rest of the way home, even up the steep hill to Bowie Court, and joined my deeply surprised mother for dinner.

Daisy moved in with our family in 1968, and she immediately became my closest friend. On game days, we would sit together listening to Washington Senator's baseball games on the radio, consoling ourselves for the usual loss with the oval delights of Russell-Stover candy. She always had a stash, because her Beau would send (for her birthday or holiday or just whenever) boxes of the assorted chocolates.

Granville Gorton Lindsay was born June 27, 1888, in King George county Virginia. He married Mary Parker in 1912, and they were married for forty-five years before Mary died in 1957.

By the 1960s, Gorton lived in Severna Park, Maryland, an hour's ride from Rockville. How or when he and Daisy reconnected after so many years I don't know. I do know my Aunt

Marg would take them on trips together down to Colonial Beach, Virginia, very near where Gorton is buried today. Once called the Playground of the Potomac, Colonial Beach is a resort town about mid-way between Washington DC and the point where the river empties into the Chesapeake Bay. In the Sixties, the town boasted a fine mile-long beach and casinos along the waterfront. I vaguely remember accompanying them, maybe by boat, since my aunt was a boater all her life.

The word Beau comes from the French word for beautiful. One of the variant connotations of the word is a man who is well dressed and well mannered. That was certainly Gorton.

Gorton when I knew him was a tall slender man, always dapper, with a brass-handled wooden cane and, often, a straw skimmer. His long strides were graceful even at his age. He was the model of a southern gentleman, always gracious, always kind, yet with a sly humor.

His manner with Daisy was more than gentlemanly; it was courtly. Even my young self thought the sight of an eighty-year-old couple walking together down the boardwalk, taking such obvious joy in one another, was completely charming. My older more knowledgeable self now remembers it as a wonder of the ancient world.

Eventually, even with the magnifying glass, she could not read the letters. So I would read them to her. I don't remember them well, except that they always opened and closed with frank expressions of his deep affection for her. I wonder sometimes if I learned then how to write to a woman, better than I have since learned to talk to one.

I have tried to remember how I felt reading the letters; I'm not sure I do. But I am pretty sure I was not embarrassed to be reading something so private, but felt bad that someone had to, that she could not read them on her own, and proud that she trusted me to do so. It was a deep sharing between us.

Gorton died in August 1970. Daisy passed just a few months later. Their moments together in their last years were brief, but still shine for me in memory.

The letters are gone too, as far as I know. I have only one fragment, a poem Gorton wrote to Daisy:

> *Lovely roses should adorn*
> *Those who in warm July are born*
> *Then will they be exempt and free*
> *From love's doubt and anxiety*
>
> *To my precious sweetheart Daisy*
> *With all my love. Gorton.*

Great hearts are never entirely lost to the world, because they have shaped it.

Daisy and Gorton shaped mine.

The Resilience of Roses

Something keeps eating my father's roses.

Or picking them, possibly. But I think likely it/they are eating them, because sometimes they also munch the new and presumably tender shoots. Probably it is the deer who frequent the green space behind me evening and morning.

I say they are my father's roses, but that is not strictly true. He passed away about five years ago. And I think my brother planted the bush in the first place. But I think of them as his, because he would often snip a blossom in the morning and have it waiting in a vase for my mother to find. Title enough, I think.

I don't really mind that something is eating the roses, though I would enjoy looking at them myself. I'm glad someone is enjoying them, and my father would have liked seeing the deer, or does like possibly--English does not have an Eternal tense.

What I enjoy as much as the sight (or memory) of the roses is the astonishing ability of the bush to regenerate itself. Hardly has one blossom fallen then another bursts forth, and the delicate leaves rush to renew.

It reminds of the lines from Spenser:

> *What though the sea with waves continuall*
> *Doe eate the earth, it is no more at all:*
> *Ne is the earth the lesse, or loseth ought,*
> *For whatsoever from one place doth fall,*
> *Is with the tide unto an other brought:*
> *For there is nothing lost, that may be found, if*
> *sought.*

I hope so.

Wren Song

I was sitting by Mom's bedside this morning. It had been hot in the room all night and we had the window cracked a bit. A wren, one of Dad's favorite birds, was sitting outside on the fence, trilling away. I was looking out the window enjoying the morning song, when on my left I thought I saw someone walk into the room. The sensation was quick, like the reflection of a headlight on a windshield.

He was tall and slender, dressed in light-colored clothing. I didn't see the face, just the form. But I had the impression it was my brother Michael, not just because the height was right, but also because of the walk. Mike had a unique walk, almost a glide, as if gravity was different where he was. I hadn't seen it since he passed away but I remembered it immediately.

When I turned my head, no one was there. Or at least: I couldn't see anyone.

But the wren kept singing, not to me.

Eulogy

When you are growing up, it's hard to see your mother as anything but Mom. And when she is riding herd on four rowdy boys, it's probably hard to be anything else.

But Mom managed. She managed to be a wonderful neighbor and friend. She managed to travel the world with Dad to places like Rome, Paris, and London, among others. She managed to care for others, through the church, by delivering meals-on-wheels with her best friend Mrs. Copeland - for close to three decades, and by making time for her special friends like Tillie Blankenship, whom she visited weekly for years.

In later years, we were privileged to spend a lot of time with her, and we began to see other sides of her. When Mom was nine years old, she lost her father, and in many ways this was the formative event of her life. It forged unbreakable bonds with her sister Margaret and her brothers Bud and Jim. It gave her the example of her own extraordinary mother

Daisy, who with grace and fortitude raised a family on her own in the midst the Great Depression. And it taught her that family is something to be protected and cherished. These are the values she taught us, the values she exemplified, in her life and in her marriage.

For much of their life together, our father rose early and our mother rose late. What role this played in the success of their 63 year marriage we can only guess.

For the last few months of his life, Dad could not stand or walk on his own. So after breakfast, he would sit in his armchair, watch old movies on TV, and wait for my mother to get up. He could see the bedroom from where he sat, and he kept a close watch for any light in the doorway.

When Mom finally appeared, he would give a loud sigh, raise his arms, and wait for his morning kiss and hug. Afterwards, he would smile his trademark smile and sink contentedly back into his chair. For the moment, despite the illnesses that had curtailed their lives, all was right.

We had the privilege of witnessing this daily moment of enduring affection. The tenderness in that simple gesture was a revelation. If anything human abides it must be this: my father keeping a keen eye, watching for the light in the doorway.

And now the door is open.

And now the light is shining.

STEPHEN EVANS

A Dream of Mom

Mom was lost and wandering, or maybe escaping from something. We took her to DuWayne's house and he said he had a bed for her upstairs. Bud and Marg were there, looking the way they did when we were growing up. I lifted Mom to put her to bed. She was so light she almost floated. Chris was there to play the guitar for her – and I said that he could always get her to sleep. As she slept Marg and Bud stayed with her to watch over her.

I have been waiting for this dream.

Liebestraum

Moments there were, when out of death, and the rebellion of the flesh, there came to you, as you took stock of yourself, a dream of love.

Thomas Mann

The Magic Mountain

We think of them, the missing ones,

Passed beyond past. Yet we would know.

Here and now if only we could ask

One simple question: Was it for love

Or for the dream of love that they endured?

STEPHEN EVANS

The Three Pietas

All-changing time now darkens what was bright,
Now ushers out of darkness into light

Horace

For much of his life, my father managed an appliance store called General Electronics at 4513 Wisconsin Avenue in Northwest Washington DC, just up the street from American University. There's a Starbucks there now I think.

They sold primarily General Electric appliances for local residents. But a large part of their business was selling appliances for export.

In DC, this was a booming market. My father knew the procurement officers from embassies, consulates, and military posts all over the world, as well as many of the staffers from foreign embassies in DC. I remember one of the staffers from the Norwegian embassy would bring us lefse from the home country, a boyhood treat Dad craved.

I worked at the store most Saturday's from age 12 or so, as did my three brothers. After a few years, I knew the electrical specs for pretty much every nation from Japan to Jordan. I wasn't as introverted then and enjoyed being on the sales floor, meeting people from all over the world, surprised to find how much they valued things I took for granted, like washing machines and refrigerators.

The General Electric company offered sales incentives, and Dad often brought home new televisions or appliances, including the microwave my mother wouldn't use at first. But their favorite incentive was travel. GE would host trips for groups of top salesmen (I suspect back then they were all men). Often the same people would go on subsequent trips, and they made some lasting friendships and stayed in touch long after my father retired.

So once every couple of years, my parents would fly off to Europe and other destinations that seemed so exotic to me. The world felt larger then, yet despite the nuclear threat of the cold war, somehow safer.

I don't remember all the places they went. Paris for sure. Madrid. Mexico City (twice I think). Acapulco. Italy. Probably others.

I could figure it out. They took hundreds of photos, now stored away in a box until I get around to digitizing. They also kept matchbooks from all their travels, and my mother bought dolls from many countries.

And they bought other souvenirs. A painting of the Madonna from Spain. A silver ring (two actually, on different trips) from a Mexican silversmith. A replica of Michelangelo's David. And three miniature marble Pietas.

I'm guessing the Italy trip was my mother's favorite. A devout Church-Every-Sunday-Sodality-On-Saturday-Make-Your-Children-Go-To-Sunday-School-Even-Though-Its-On-Monday Catholic, she must have been enthralled by Rome. She visited the Vatican, saw the Sistine Chapel, had an audience with the pope (John or Paul, I'm not sure which) (and I don't mean Beatles). And bought three copies of the Pieta, Michaelangelo's statue depicting Mary holding the body of Jesus.

They are sitting side by side now in the china cabinet, with the other curios she assembled, like the girl and puppy porcelain statue I have written about elsewhere. The Pietas differ in size by maybe half an inch, and have slightly different shades of white, from snow to cream. Perhaps the color has aged, or the marble is just different.

I have often wondered why she bought three. I never thought to ask while she was alive. Did she intend them as gifts? Did she plan to give them to her four sons? (I got the David, so maybe the three Pietas were for the others, who obviously needed more spiritual help).Did she want to help the artists who carved them? Or was she just so overwhelmed by the spiritual experience?

I don't know. I'll never know I suppose. The three pietas will always be a mystery, unless she was right in her belief, and we will all be together someday, and I can ask her. It would be like her to think that far ahead. She was a great planner, with a wry sense of humor. I can see her smiling as she bought them, thinking of how puzzled I would be many years later.

If she was right, one day (or no day) I will know the answer. And be overwhelmed by the spiritual experience myself.

Yet, in some sense, it is the wondering that I crave. Keats had a phrase, negative capability, the willingness to live (and create) in a state of irreducible not knowing. In a state of wonder.

Those who reduce belief to a kind of knowing may be missing this point: the gift of wonder is the essential condition of religion, of art, maybe of sentient life, essential because it impels us forward, closer to that now unreachable truth.

So I wonder about those three pietas. I do wonder.

Keyboard

For the last few months I have been going through boxes I had in storage, some for almost two decades. One of the boxes I found had some music in it and I have started playing the piano again, a little.

Rodgers and Hart. Jerome Kern. Sigmund Romberg. I am not that old (quite), but it is my period, musically. At heart I am a balladeer.

I was never a very good musician and I am much worse now. The piano belonged to my grandmother Daisy. She was amazing, could play anything by ear alone, an early compensation for her blindness in later life.

I did not inherit my grandmother's talent. Nor my grandfather's talent with the violin. Nor my father's ability to harmonize. I did inherit my mother's talent for listening, and enjoying.

Playing again, whatever the quality, has brought some of the joy back. For one, it's a good break from that other imperious keyboard. And it's nice to know we can rediscover at any age.

Now I wonder what is in the next box.

A Christmas Card to God

I was cleaning out Mom's dresser for donations and found some worn sheets of typed correspondence in the bottom of one of the drawers. This is what they said :

Dear Lord,
    It is almost your birthday and while I have been going crazy trying to think of everyone else and what to get them, I have almost completely neglected to concentrate on a gift to you - almost. This will be my Christmas card to you, since I have just mailed all my others and can think about what I want to say to you. And guess what, as usual I find I am at a complete loss of words. As you know I have never been much of a talker but I do have very deep feelings for many things - or I should say people. I go to a nursing

home and deliver meals on wheels and I see the pain and sadness when these people are neglected. A visit means so much to them and it really doesn't cost anything but a small amount of time.

You know what is in my heart, Dear Lord, I can't con you. So, instead of giving you a gift, once again I'm asking a favor of you. Give me the grace to treat people as you would if you were here on earth, also, let me set an example for my children and husband to that they may one day find you, and as the priest said, if they don't find you - please, you find them. I must try to get to Mass more often. I always manage to go when I need some favor but I want to go more just to please you.

Well, all for now Dear Lord. Except to wish you a very happy Birthday, tune in this station next year, if still here, and see if I have improved any, in order to give you a little better birthday present then.

Love,
You know who.

Friends

I don't know how my mother came to choose the little blue house at 7 Bowie Court. But in choosing it, she changed her life, and the lives of her children.

From 1957 to 1967, we lived in that house. The Copelands were next door at 5 Bowie Court. And unlike the other houses in the court, our front doors faced each other. That access and proximity facilitated a friendship between my mother and Mrs. Copeland that lasted almost 60 years, a relationship that continued and even grew in closeness after we moved across town. As I grew up, and after, they taught me what friendship meant.

Somehow, despite (or because of?) raising seven boys between them, they seemed constant companions. This included 20 plus years or so swimming in the mornings at the Rockville Pool and 35 years of Meals in Wheels (my Mom driving, Mrs. Copeland delivering).

My mother loved to drive and Mrs. Copeland loved to explore, and they took countless trips together, usually just afternoon drives out into the country (there was country then) or up to Westminster for tea. One very special trip they both talked about for years after: down to Asheville North Carolina and over the mountains to Gatlinburg Tennessee. It was one of the things that my mother remembered longest.

Mrs. Copeland (I never could call her Ann) loved music and the arts, and had a fine soprano voice. She would frequently accompany my parents to my performances in Annapolis or elsewhere, and was well known to my performing friends. She had a discerning ear, but was effusive with her praise. When I turned to writing, she was just as supportive. And with her generous heart and love of arts and beauty, she was a continuing inspiration.

After Mom died, Mrs. Copeland would continue to call us, always apologizing for not calling sooner, asking how we were, deflecting our questions about her health, encouraging me to write, and always with the spirit and warmth and humor we had known all our lives. We have now lost a cherished presence, and a link to our past. But for me, the memory and lessons of their friendship will not fade before I do.

The Blue Cap

She wears a dark blue raincoat on this cloudy day, and a lighter blue cap, something out of the sixties. I can imagine her then, a young woman, wearing one to a party, dazzling with her golden hair and brilliant smile, charming them all.

Now her hair is white.

And white tennis shoes.

Always the white shoes.

And alone.

Always alone.

Except for the dog.

Her dog is smallish and also white, like most of the dogs in this community. For some reason, they are the canine of choice, maybe because they don't eat much or fit just so on an eighty-year old lap.

As she walks, she sways side to side. Maybe her hips don't work as they used to or she is shielding her knees. Still she walks. Twice a day. Every day. At a good pace relatively. Holding tight to the leash. As though something about it keeps her upright.

I walk past her and smile, saying Good Afternoon. She doesn't seem to recognize me, though we have passed a few times before. Her face brightens and she smiles, but she doesn't speak back. Unused now to speaking to anyone, except her children on the phone every few weeks.

She is alone. Always alone. Except for the dog, who is now the beneficiary of all the love and care she has stored up since her husband passed.

So she walks every day. Rain or shine. In peril of falling every step it seems to me. I worry for her.

She is alone. Yet there are many like her here in this community. She passes them every day. They have never spoken yet they know each other.

As she passes me, I turn and watch for a second.

Maybe this is not her story. Maybe she has a family close to her, who visit most days, like my next door neighbor. Maybe her husband does the laundry and she walks the dog for exercise. I don't really know.

But as I imagine her, she is a reminder. And a warning. And an inspiration.

Go find my blue cap.

An Observation

It isn't grief that leaves you.

It's the memory of grief.

Bloom

I have written before about the resilience of the rose bush behind my apartment. But between the deer last year and the late freezes this year, I think the rose bush has finally met its match. As you can guess, I am sad about it.

There is an azalea bush next to the rose bush, and, if I recall rightly (always a question these days), it was planted for my mother by my brother Michael nearly fifteen years ago, not long after they moved in here. In all those years to my knowledge it never bloomed.

I am no gardener, but I often wondered if it wasn't getting enough sun, or rain. But maybe it was just waiting for the right moment.

Both Mike and Mom are gone now, but I hope they are watching from heaven, because their azalea has bloomed for the first time, two beautiful pink blossoms.

I guess you never know what is going to bloom.

Or when.

Kintsugi

Kintsugi（金継ぎ）is the Japanese art of repairing broken items with gold. The gold highlights the area of the breakage, with the idea that the history of the object is part of its beauty. My father practiced his own version of Kintsugi, though not with gold. Exactly.

My mother owned a small porcelain statue of a girl and a puppy, a Hummel or something like. It is an endearing image, or it was originally. With four boys and a continuing series of dogs in the house, that poor little girl endured many accidents during the fifty or so years she has graced our presence. The puppy somehow escaped mostly unscathed.

My mother loved the statue. So every time it was broken, my father brought out the Elmer's glue and painstakingly tried to put her back together. I can't begin to count the number of times, or ever forget the image of my 6' 4'' (and a half he would insist, just like John Wayne) father hunched over the table with his calloused hands tracing the delicate porcelain pieces with a toothpick, painstakingly applying the white adhesive.

The result was never perfect, or even close. Seams are visible everywhere. Some parts never fit back together right. Some are gone completely. But it is still Kintsugi to me—the mending preserves their history together. The gold is in the memory.

The statue now sits on the top shelf of my china cabinet, safely keeping company with other vestiges of that era. I think sometimes of giving her away. But I haven't. I can't. Who but me will see the decades of love melded in the mending? Who but me?

Yet now, we.

And that is mending too.

The Narrowing

As I turn 65, I am increasingly aware of a Narrowing in my life, the sense that the parameters, the boundaries, have closed in, and will continue to do so. My life, which had been a pyramid, has become a pillar. I am the atlas alone atop the stone, bearing the weight of the decisions that have placed me here

It makes sense in a way. The narrowing may have started soon after the most notable widening of my life. In 1993, I moved to Minneapolis. My wife and I had started our marriage in Washington DC, which was home to me. But she hated the traffic and her job and possibly me. So we decided to move to Minneapolis, her home of many years. I had hoped the move might rescue the marriage, but it didn't. It did open my eyes in other ways, though, as moving someplace new can do. And Minneapolis, despite or because of the grand disruption of my life and plans, Minneapolis with its lakes and arts and smiling people, opened my creative heart, and the city became a muse.

My mind, which had always been pretty open, waited for its own muse, and it was not long in coming. In 1997, after the marriage had ended in the mutual recognition that we had engaged in hopes unfounded in reality or personality, I took a solo car trip across country, a transcendental journey described elsewhere. This was I think the widest moment of my life, where any road seemed open to me, reaching its apex on a highway on the plains of South Dakota, as the limits of the world fell away, the road went on forever, and the moment was defined by freedom.

But as I discovered on that trip, in choosing one road, others are let go. In the year or two that followed, I chose two roads. I chose to be a writer, and I chose to take care of family.

I see now (though I did not completely at the time) that in making those choices I let others go. Marriage or any kind of romantic partnership was not included. Deep friendships in essence became infrequent companions in practice. No one asked me to make these choices. I made them, and I don't question the choices now, because they seemed best to me then, and what good would it do anyway? Focus and necessity became my principles, though perhaps they were only a cover. Perhaps the Narrowing had already begun.

My choices came with a cost, and that cost has become the Narrowing. My life is circumscribed into smaller and smaller limits. A trip to the store or Starbucks is my adventure for the day. I dream of travel, but the effort and stress and uncertainty seem beyond my powers. I don't drive at night, or on the highway, or to places I don't know. I have lived in this apartment for nearly twenty years, not because I like it (though for the most part I do), but because the thought of uprooting my life at this age, and from within this solitude, is daunting.

I watched this Narrowing towards the end of my parents life. Once world travelers, wonderful friends, wide readers, their world became chair and bed, television and tray, doctor and hospital. I live in a retirement community and I see daily that my life is not the only one Narrowed. Many others around me have been, by grief, by isolation, by illness, by money, by age itself.

The Narrowing in my case is based less on capacity than on fear. I see this. But so far I have not been able to work past it. As an intelligent person, I feel that I should be able to. I should be able to solve this problem. And sometimes I feel that I am on the brink. I am not sure of what—a widening, reformation, a renaissance? So far the brink is as far as I have reached.

Yet other times, as I sit in my chair and listen to music or read or write, I have a vision I can only dimly apprehend, like the Xanadu of Coleridge (without the opium), a vague sense that the Narrowing is in its own way a transition to be embraced.

As the pyramid narrows into the pillar, the atlas atop climbs higher. The base is more unsteady, and toppling is a twist away. But the scene is expansive. We see farther, and further. Beyond ourselves.

And as the clouds dissipate, the view is transcendent.

My Mother's Angels

My mother collected angels. She found and brought them home from all over. Now that she has passed, I have been trying to decide what to do with them.

Some at least I will keep: the brass candle holders she bought in Mexico, and definitely the musical one that chimes *Hark the Herald Angels Sing* when you wind it.

I was not healthy as a child, asthma that kept me indoors for weeks, whole months of school missed, severe bouts of pneumonia. During these, according to my father, there were times when he did not think I would make it. I don't remember that.

But I do remember my mother sitting with me through the night, night after night, as I struggled to breathe, vaporizer on full blast, cooling my fever and reading to me to keep me calm and entertained. Most clearly I remember her reading *Winnie the Pooh* and *The House at Pooh Corner*, doing all the voices. I still hear her voice when I read them. And I still read them to hear her voice.

So some of the angels I think I will let go, in the hope that they may carry into the world the gifts that she gave me. The gift of presence.

The gift of care.

The gift of example.

The gift of knowing every day that you are loved.

If anyone can carry these gifts, it will be my mother's angels.

Index

STEPHEN EVANS

Acknowledgements

Many of these pieces appeared first on The Green Room (www.gr8word.com).

Harpman was the title of a poem written and read at Mike's wake by his friend Charlie Shapira.

I have been so fortunate in my life to grow up and just grow with my family and friends. I am grateful to them all.

About the Author

Stephen Evans is a playwright and the author of A Transcendental Journey, Painting Sunsets, and The Island of Always. Find him online at:

https://www.istephenevans.com/

https://www.facebook.com/iStephenEvans

https://twitter.com/iStephenEvans

STEPHEN EVANS

STEPHEN EVANS

STEPHEN EVANS

Lightning Source UK Ltd.
Milton Keynes UK
UKHW010810111220
374897UK00002B/429